Hand
Inter

Merry Christmas
to BMH ER
Early
1991

Handbook of Pediatric ECG Interpretation

WILLIAM BERMAN, JR., M.D.
Pediatric Cardiology Associates of
New Mexico
Adjunct Professor of Pediatrics
University of New Mexico
School of Medicine
Albuquerque, New Mexico

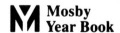
Mosby
Year Book

St. Louis   Baltimore   Boston   Chicago   London   Philadelphia   Sydney   Toronto

**Mosby
Year Book**

Dedicated to Publishing Excellence

Sponsoring Editor: Don Ladig
Developmental Editor: Winifred Sullivan
Associate Managing Editor, Manuscript Services:
Deborah Thorp
Production Coordinator: Nancy C. Baker
Proofroom Manager: Barbara Kelly

Mosby-Year Book, Inc.
11830 Westline Industrial Drive
St. Louis, MO 63146

1   2   3   4   5   6   7   8   9   0   CL/MA   95
                    94   93   92   91

FOREWORD

The two most valuable commodities needed by a busy clinician are knowledge and time. This manual offers the former without wasting the latter. Pediatric acute care providers spend a significant amount of time recording and examining ECG rhythm strips, yet often lack a fundamental knowledge of ECG interpretation. Although several extensive reference texts are available, the bedside clinician has no time to consult such material. This pocket reference provides a succinct review of essential aspects of pediatric ECG interpretation; it leads the reader from the fundamentals through interpretation of dysrhythmias with plenty of illustrations and tables. This book will undoubtedly prove to be a valuable resource for the busy bedside nurse and resident physician.

The advanced pediatric life support course from the American Heart Association emphasized the importance of three dysrhythmias in pediatric patients: bradyarrhythmias, tachyarrhythmias, and collapse rhythms. The *Handbook of Pediatric ECG Interpretation* builds on this information while retaining its emphasis on essential dysrhythmias. Chapter 4, Disorders of Rate and Rhythm, will be most valuable to the bedside clinician; it is filled with practical hints and methods of distinguishing significant from benign rhythms.

This manual should be read through in its entirety, since every chapter contains valuable, practical information. However, the clear division of material in the book and short chapter format are ideal for "quick reference" at the bedside. Dr. Berman is a skilled teacher and cardiologist, and he has distilled pediatric ECG interpretation to its essence.

Mary Fran Hazinski, R.N., M.S.N., F.A.A.N.

PREFACE

"The little less, and what worlds away"
Thomas Hardy

The "world" hardly needs another extensive treatise on ECG interpretation. This is not meant to be that. It is, instead, a working manual: brief, scantily referenced, and heavily reliant on personal experience. It is directed to primary care providers for infants and children, including pediatricians and family practitioners, medical students, house staff, and nurses. The tracings are stylized and simplified to illustrate text points more clearly. Much of the foundation for what follows was laid by Paul Stanger, M.D., of San Francisco and Steve Yabek, M.D., of Albuquerque; they are in no way to be held accountable, however, for the final product.

William Berman, Jr., M.D.

CONTENTS

THE WAVE
FORMS AND
INTERVALS

1

Accurate ECG interpretation is dependent on recognition and analysis of each of the components of the tracing. In this section, the wave forms which contribute to the ECG are reviewed briefly.

When analyzing any ECG deflection, it is important to point out that the size and configuration of the deflection are affected by the direction from which the electrical events are viewed. Accordingly, points of observation along the electrical axis of a deflection will yield waves which are larger (in either a positive or negative direction) than deflections viewed from observation points more nearly perpendicular to the axis of the wave form. For purpose of review, the ECG leads in the frontal and coronal planes are depicted in Figure 1–1,A through C.

As one can see, the standard limb leads (I,II,III) and augmented limb leads (aVR,aVL,aVF) describe the electrical activation pattern in the frontal plane, whereas the chest (also called precordial) leads— including leads V_3R, V_4R, and V_7—describe the electrical events in the coronal plane. From the dia-

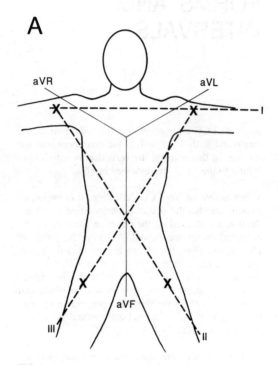

FIG 1-1.
A, limb ECG lead placement. *Continued*.

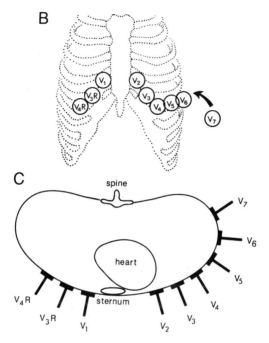

FIG 1–1 (cont.).
B, precordial ECG lead placement. **C,** precordial ECG leads in coronal plane.

grams, one can see that an ECG wave with a frontal plane axis of +60 degrees will give a deflection which is highest (and, therefore, often most easy to interpret) in lead II in the frontal plane. Similarly, in the coronal plane, electrical forces directed anteriorly will cause large deflections in leads V_1 and

V_2, but little deflection in lead V_6; leftward forces, however, will cause prominent deflections in lead V_6, but not in leads V_1 and V_2. This relationship between the point of observation and the tracing obtained makes some leads more useful than others for the diagnosis of atrial enlargement and ventricular hypertrophy. It also makes it essential that more than one lead be viewed in the analysis of cardiac arrhythmias, as wave form patterns that are obvious in one lead may be obscure, absent, or uninterpretable in other leads.

RATES AND INTERVALS

The ECG tracing is recorded usually at a rate of 25 mm/sec. Occasionally, a "paper speed" of 50 mm/sec is used to facilitate interval measurement or wave form interpretation. At the standard rate of 25 mm/sec, as one can see from Fig 1–2, each millimeter box horizontally represents a time interval of 0.04 second; each *emphasized* 5-mm box corresponds to a time interval of 0.2 second. These markers are required for wave form analysis and interval calculation. Also, they can be used to quantify heart rate, *if* the rate is regular:

5-mm Box Interval	R-R Interval (sec)	Heart Rate (b pm)
1	0.2	300
2	0.4	150
3	0.6	100
4	0.8	75
5	1.0	60
6	1.2	50

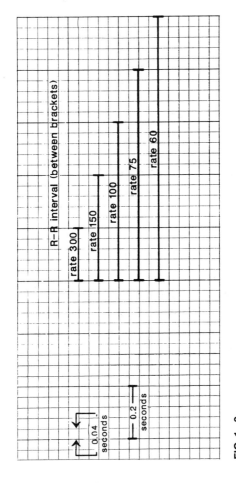

FIG 1–2.
Heart rate calculation at normal (25 mm/sec) paper speed.

THE P WAVE (ATRIAL DEPOLARIZATION)

The P wave normally has a frontal plane axis between +30 and +90 degrees. The P wave originates normally from the sinus node, which lies at the junction of the superior vena cava and the right atrium, and proceeds from right to left across the atria. In the coronal plane, right atrial forces are directed anteriorly and left atrial forces both posteriorly and to the left. The P wave is a "composite" wave form, consisting of components originating from both the right and left atria (Fig 1–3).

The right atrial deflection precedes the left, as one would expect from the discussion above. The P wave, then, is the electrical summation of these two component parts. These factors make the diagnosis of atrial enlargement, as described in Chapter 2, more understandable.

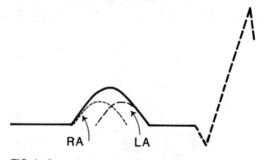

FIG 1–3.
Right *(RA)* and left *(LA)* atrial contributions to composite P wave.

THE QRS COMPLEX (VENTRICULAR DEPOLARIZATION)

The QRS complex reflects depolarization of the interventricular septum and both ventricles. Normally, the electrical activation of this portion of the heart proceeds from the AV node to the inferior and left side of the interventricular septum. The septal depolarization from left to right, in a superior direction, is the first (earliest) event in the QRS complex; it represents the Q wave seen in the left precordial (chest) leads of the normal ECG. The remainder of the QRS deflection reflects depolarization of the right and left ventricles.

The nomenclature of this wave form can be confusing:

- A Q wave refers to an *initial* negative deflection.
- An R wave is the first positive deflection.
- An S wave is a negative deflection *following* a positive deflection.

Lower-case and capital letters are used to denote the size of the components of the wave form relative to one another; a lower-case letter refers to a small deflection and a capital letter to a large one. In addition, in tracings containing two or more R and/or S waves, a prime sign is used to distinguish subsequent from initial deflections. In Figure 1–4,a on the facing page, the correct description would be qRs; in Figure 1–4,b, RS; in Figure 1–4,c, rSR'.

The size, axis, and configuration of the QRS complex are useful for the diagnosis of ventricular hy-

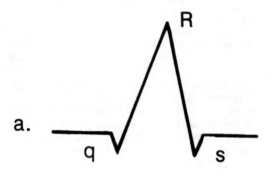

a.

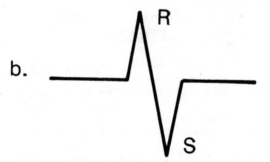

b.

FIG 1-4.
QRS nomenclature. *Continued.*

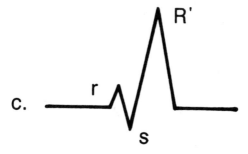

FIG 1–4   (cont.).

pertrophy, as described in Chapter 3. Normally, the overall axis of the QRS deflection is more rightward at birth than it is later in life. The range of normal for QRS axis is broad and summarized in Table 1–1.

The axis of any wave form can be determined most easily by finding the lead in which the wave form is most nearly isoelectric, that is to say, the *area* under the positive deflection and that under the negative deflection are most nearly equal. In Figure 1–5, *both* wave forms a and b are isoelectric, whereas wave form c is not.

Once the isoelectric lead is determined, the leads at or nearly at right angles to that lead are examined to determine the direction of the electrical axis. In Figure 1–6 (p. 13), a wave form is isoelectric in lead II (+60 degrees). The axis of this wave form could be −30 degrees or +150 degrees, that is, in a direction

TABLE 1–1.

Guidelines for ECG Interpretation*

Variable	1 Day	1–3 mo	6–9 mo	1–2 yr	3–10 yr	>10 yr
Resting heart rate (bpm)						
90th percentile	170	185	155	135	125	100
Average	125	150	135	120	100	85
10th percentile	100	105	100	90	70	?55?
Sleeping—lower limit of normal	80	80	70	70	60	50
QRS axis (degrees)						
90th percentile	170	110	100	90	80	80
Average	132	73	64	61	54	56
10th percentile	110	30	30	20	10	20
PR interval (sec); upper limits of normal at heart rate of:						
70 bpm						.18
71–90 bpm	.11					.18
91–110 bpm	.11	.14	.14	.15	.16	.16
111–130 bpm	.11	.13	.14	.14	.16	.16
131–150 bpm	.11	.12	.12	.14	.15	.16
>151 bpm		.11	.11	.12		

*Modified from Gillette PC, Garson A Jr: *Pediatric Arrhythmias: Electrophysiology and Pacing,* ed 9. Philadelphia, WB Saunders Co, 1990, p 252.

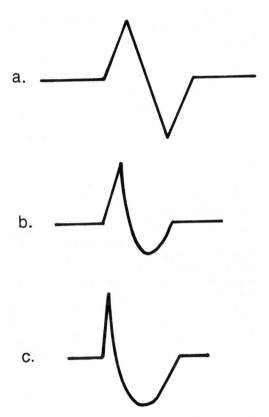

FIG 1–5.
"Isoelectric" deflections (**a** and **b**); net negative deflection (**c**).

perpendicular to the isoelectric lead. To make the distinction, one views leads aVL and III; in Fig 1–6 one can see an overall negative deflection in aVL and a positive one in III. The axis, therefore, is +150 degrees.

When the axis of depolarization is between two leads (as in Fig 1–7 where the axis falls between II and aVF, between +60 and +90 degrees), by convention the axis is assigned an angle halfway between the two leads, in this case, +75 degrees.

THE T WAVE (VENTRICULAR REPOLARIZATION)

Normally, the T wave axis is similar to the QRS axis because of two cellular electrical factors: cellular repolarization causes a deflection opposite in direction to cellular depolarization, *but* ventricular repolarization occurs in a sequence opposite to that of depolarization. Therefore, although the direction of repolarization is opposite to that of depolarization, the cellular (and, therefore, ECG) electrical forces are reversed, resulting in a T wave axis similar to that of the QRS complex. After the first few months of life, if the T wave axis differs by more than 60 degrees from the axis of the QRS complex, there is said to be QRS-T discordance, a repolarization abnormality often indicative of ventricular strain or hypertrophy.

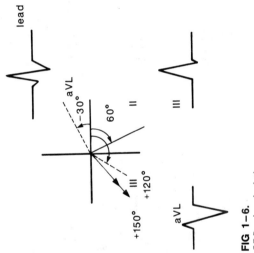

FIG 1–6.
QRS axis calculation.

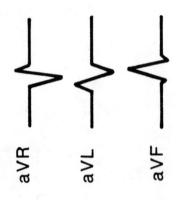

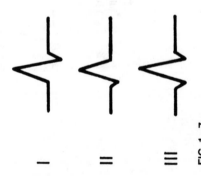

FIG 1–7.
QRS axis +75 degrees.

THE PR INTERVAL

The interval in time between the *onset* of the P wave and the *onset* of the QRS complex is termed the *PR interval* (Fig 1–8).

The PR interval varies with both age and heart rate. The higher the heart rate, the shorter the PR interval; for a given rate, the younger the age, the shorter the PR interval. From Table 1–1, which relates the upper limit of normal for the PR interval to both age and heart rate, one can see that a PR interval of 0.14 second is normal for a 2-year-old with a heart rate of 110 bpm, but prolonged for a newborn with the same rate. Additionally, that same PR interval would be prolonged for the 2-year-old during exercise and a heart rate of 165 bpm. Other examples can be created by the reader. Relative prolongation of the PR interval constitutes the diagnostic criterion for first degree heart block, as discussed in Chapter 4; in contrast, a short PR interval suggests aberrant atrial to ventricular conduction, as in the WPW syndrome, also discussed in Chapter 4.

QRS DURATION

Normally, the activation of the ventricular septum and ventricles occurs in less than 0.1 second. A QRS duration over 0.09 seconds in infants and children under age 3 years; over 0.10 seconds in children 3 to 12 years old; and over 0.12 seconds in adolescents and young adults constitutes the diagnostic criterion for bundle-branch block, that is, pathologic slowing of conduction through one of the bundle branches. When conduction is interrupted entirely in

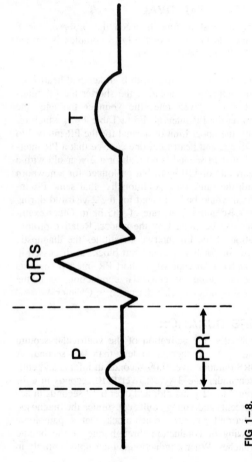

FIG 1–8.
PR interval.

a bundle branch, a shift in frontal plane QRS axis usually occurs as a leftward shift with interruption of the anterior division of the left bundle branch. The site of slowed or blocked conduction is reflected as well by the morphology of the QRS complex in the frontal and coronal planes. Terminal "slowing" of conduction occurs because the electrical impulse is passing directly through muscle rather than conducting tissue. Slowed conduction over the right chest leads reflects right bundle-branch block, whereas slowed conduction over the left chest leads reflects left bundle-branch block (Fig 1–9).

When conduction through the ventricles is tortuous, but the duration of the QRS complex does not meet criteria for bundle-branch block, a diagnosis of ventricular *conduction delay* is made. This is often represented by an rSR' deflection pattern, resulting in turn from a figure-of-eight vector loop through the ventricles, rather than the usual elliptical loop pattern (Marriott, 1983).

Intraventricular conduction delays may be normal, result from a volume overload of the ventricle (*right* ventricular conduction delay is usual with ASD), or may reflect drug effects or electrolyte abnormalities (*left* ventricular conduction delay and even bundle-branch block has been seen in premature infants with hyperkalemia).

THE QT INTERVAL

The interval between the *onset* of the QRS complex and the *end* of the T wave is referred to as the *QT interval* (Fig 1–10).

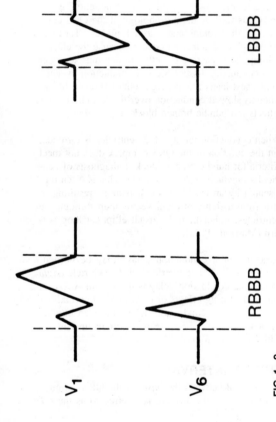

FIG 1–9.
QRS configurations in *right (RBBB)* and *left (LBBB)* bundle-branch block.

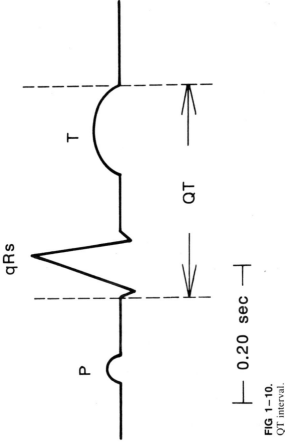

FIG 1–10.
QT interval.

The QT interval is affected by heart rate, shortening normally at more rapid rates and lengthening at slower rates. For this reason, the QT interval is best "corrected" for rate, by referencing it to a rate of 60 bpm. This is done by dividing the absolute QT interval by the square root of the interval in seconds between R waves (that is, the cycle length). For a heart rate of 60 bpm, the cycle length is 1 second, the square root of which is 1; the corrected QT interval (QT_c) and the absolute QT interval are the same. With cycle lengths less than 1 second (rates over 60 bpm), the square root term is less than 1 and the QT_c exceeds the absolute QT measurement. For heart rates under 60 bpm, the converse is true. The normal range of QT_c intervals may vary with age as well as heart rate (Schwartz et al., 1982; Ahnve, 1985). For subjects beyond the newborn period, a QT_c of 0.45 second or more is prolonged.

The QT interval is modulated by the autonomic nervous system, and affected by a variety of electrolyte, mineral, and acid-base disorders. The most common causes of QT_c interval prolongation in pediatrics are hypocalcemia and/or hypomagnesemia associated with perinatal asphyxia, and hypokalemia. In addition, two different hereditary syndromes thought to involve imbalance of the laterality of the autonomic system are associated with QT_c interval prolongation and the risk of syncope, neurologic complications, or sudden death from ventricular tachyarrhythmias: the Jervell and Lange-Nielsen syndrome is associated with nerve deafness and is an autosomal recessive trait; and the Romano-Ward syndrome is associated with normal hearing, and is transmitted by autosomal dominant inheritance with variable penetrance (Schwartz et al., 1975).

NOTES

NOTES

ATRIAL ENLARGEMENT

2

The atrial activation sequence described in Chapter 1 provides the basis for diagnosis of atrial enlargement on the ECG. Because the findings to be described can occur with atrial distension due to acute changes in ventricular compliance or afterload (in the absence of any hypertrophy of the atrial wall), pathologic findings in the P wave form are by convention said to represent atrial *enlargement* rather than atrial hypertrophy.

RIGHT ATRIAL ENLARGEMENT

With enlargement or distension of the right atrium, the initial portion (right atrial contribution) of the P wave tracing is increased in amplitude and duration (see the box on common causes of RAE). However, the duration increase of the right atrial component does not affect the overall duration of the composite P wave, which remains less than 0.08 seconds long. Because of the increased amplitude of the right atrial component, the P wave can assume a tall and peaked configuration. With a normal P wave axis in the range of +60 degrees, these changes are viewed best in the frontal plane in lead II. A P wave in lead II with a peaked configuration and a height over 2.5

COMMON CAUSES OF RIGHT ATRIAL ENLARGEMENT

Increased volume

High systemic output (AV fistula—as hepatic or cerebral, endocrine disorders)

Tricuspid incompetence (in newborn, Ebstein's anomaly, endocardial cushion defect, post cardiac surgery)

Abnormal communications (pulmonary venous drainage anomalies, sinus of Valsalva to right atrium fistula)

Rhythm disorders (following termination of SVT, third degree AV block with bradycardia)

Increased pressure

Tricuspid stenosis or atresia

Right ventricular hypertension (as transposition of the great vessels or pulmonary atresia)

Pulmonary artery hypertension (large VSD or PDA, pulmonary vascular obstructive disease)

---

mm at full standard tracing conditions satisfies criteria for the diagnosis of right atrial enlargement (Fig 2–1).

Changes may be apparent also in the anterior coronal plane chest leads, V_1 and V_2, where the P wave pattern again is tall and peaked, but not broad.

LEFT ATRIAL ENLARGEMENT

With LAE, the terminal forces of the P wave are increased in amplitude and duration (see box for com-

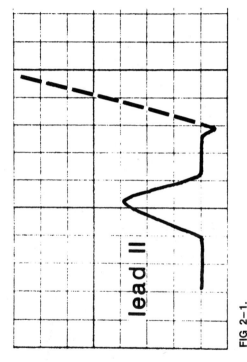

FIG 2–1.
Right atrial enlargement.

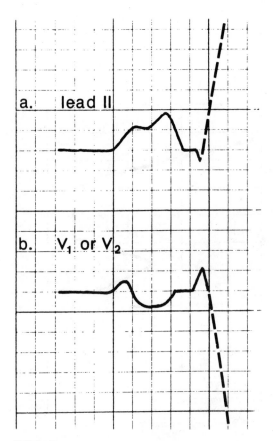

FIG 2-2.
Left atrial enlargement.

COMMON CAUSES OF LEFT ATRIAL ENLARGEMENT

Increased volume
  High pulmonary blood flow with an intact
    atrial septum (VSD, PDA, aortopulmonary
    shunts)
  Mitral incompetence (rheumatic, mitral valve
    prolapse, endocardial cushion defect)
Increased pressure
  Mitral stenosis
  Left ventricular outflow tract obstruction (aor-
    tic stenosis, subaortic stenosis, coarctation)
  Systemic hypertension

---

mon causes of LAE). Because it is the terminal section of the P wave that is affected by LAE, the
duration of the P wave increases, usually to exceed
0.1 seconds. Moreover, the second component of
the P wave is more prominent than is normally the
case, and therefore, again in frontal plane limb lead
II, the P wave may take on a notched or double-
humped appearance (Fig 2–2,a). When viewed
from the anterior chest leads, left atrial activation is
a posterior phenomenon. Accordingly, in leads V_1
and V_2, LAE appears as a P wave which is *prolonged* in duration and biphasic in configuration,
with a small initial positive deflection (the right
atrial component) and a slurred and prolonged terminal negative deflection (Fig 2–2,b).

NOTES

NOTES

VENTRICULAR HYPERTROPHY

3

The diagnosis of ventricular hypertrophy is a common focus of pediatric ECG interpretation. In the immediate perinatal period, there is a physiologic dominance of right ventricular forces, evidenced by a relative rightward frontal plane axis of the QRS complex (see Table 1–1), prominent positive deflections in the anterior chest leads, and prominent negative deflections in the left chest leads. As will become evident from the discussion, at any age the diagnosis of RVH is more straightforward than the diagnosis of LVH.

RIGHT VENTRICULAR HYPERTROPHY

For diagnosis of RVH (see box for common causes of RVH), the augmented limb lead aVR and the anterior chest leads (V_4R, V_3R, and V_1) are most useful. The diagnosis of right ventricular hypertrophy can be distilled into four elements:

1. An R wave in aVR over 5 mm suggests RVH.

2. A qR pattern in the anterior chest leads is diagnostic of RVH, at *any* age. In making this diagnosis, the qR pattern must be distinguished carefully

COMMON CAUSES OF RIGHT VENTRICULAR
HYPERTROPHY

Increased volume
  Shunts at the atrial level (ASD, anomalous
    pulmonary venous drainage)
  Valvar incompetence (tricuspid or pulmonic)
Increased pressure
  Right ventricular outflow tract obstruction
    (pulmonic stenosis, subpulmonic stenosis,
    tetralogy of Fallot, peripheral pulmonic
    stenosis, obstructed pulmonary venous
    drainage)
  Pulmonary artery hypertension
    Secondary to communicating lesions (VSD,
      PDA, endocardial cushion defect)
    Secondary to elevated pulmonary vascular
      resistance (altitude, pulmonary vascular
      obstructive disease, chronic hypoxemia,
      bronchopulmonary dysplasia)
  Miscellaneous—coarctation of the aorta in
    the *newborn*

from an rSR′ pattern with a very small initial r wave
(Fig 3–1).
3. After 2 weeks of age, an *isolated* R wave in the
right chest leads is diagnostic of RVH. Again the
isolated R wave must be distinguished carefully
from an Rs pattern (Fig 3–2).
4. Finally, careful attention must be paid to T wave
morphology in the anterior chest leads. At or near
the time of birth, the T wave in the right chest leads
becomes positive in amplitude. In most neonates,

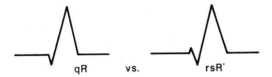

FIG 3–1.
qR vs. rSR' pattern.

this pattern changes normally to a negative deflection by 5 days of age, but in some subjects this change may not occur until 10 days of age. Sometime between 6 years of age and adulthood, T waves in the right chest leads most often become positive again. Physiologically, then, between 10 days and 6 years of age, T waves in the right chest leads are inverted. If the T waves in V_4R, V_3R, and V_1 are flat or upright between these age limits, a repolarization abnormality exists and is reflective of RVH. It is a pattern parallel to flat or inverted T waves in the left chest leads, a finding strongly suggestive of LVH. Repolarizations are affected by digitalis and, consequently, one cannot use T wave criteria for diagnosis of ventricular hypertrophy in patients receiving any form of that drug.

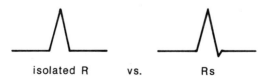

FIG 3–2.
Isolated R wave vs. Rs pattern.

LEFT VENTRICULAR HYPERTROPHY

Criteria for the diagnosis of LVH are less well defined and agreed upon:

1. An S wave deflection greater than 15 mm in lead aVR is suggestive of LVH.

2. The height of the R wave in chest lead V_6 is useful in the diagnosis of LVH. The upper limit of normal for R wave amplitude in V_6 is 10 mm in the newborn, 15 mm in the 10-day-old, 20 mm in the 3- to 4-month-old, and 22 mm in the 9-month-old. Little change in the upper limit of normal occurs beyond age 9 months. Therefore, an R wave amplitude in V_6 of 23 mm or more in a subject over 9 months of age satisfies voltage criteria for the diagnosis of LVH.

3. T wave flattening or inversion in the left chest leads (V_6 and V_7) is strongly suggestive of LVH. This repolarization abnormality, often associated with depression or elevation of the ST segment of the ECG, may result from drug effect (as digoxin), electrolyte disturbance, or pericardial inflammation. As in adults, however, it may reflect myocardial ischemia, which can occur in children with severe aortic stenosis, anomalous origin of the left coronary artery, or structural coronary disease secondary to Kawasaki's syndrome or rejection following cardiac transplantation (see box on causes of LVH).

4. Unfortunately, LVH does not always occur in a leftward direction. Leftward LVH causes the classic large negative deflection in lead aVR and the large positive deflections in the left chest leads. However, LVH may also occur in *inferior* and *posterior* direc-

---

COMMON CAUSES OF LEFT VENTRICULAR
HYPERTROPHY

Increased volume
    Left-to-right shunts distal to the left atrium
        (VSD, PDA, following aortopulmonary
        shunts, tricuspid atresia with VSD, etc.)
    Mitral valve incompetence (mitral valve pro-
        lapse, endocardial cushion defect, rheu-
        matic)
    Aortic valve incompetence (post cardiac sur-
        gery, rheumatic, post SBE)
    High output states
    Chronic bradycardia
Increased pressure
    Left ventricular outflow tract obstruction (AS,
        sub-AS, coarctation)
    Systemic hypertension
Myopathy—obstructive or congestive (idio-
    pathic, postinfectious, anomalous origin of
    the left coronary artery)
miscellaneous—glycogen storage disease type
    IIa (Pompe's)

---

tions. Inferior LVH causes prominent R waves in
the inferior limb leads II, III, and aVF (Fig
3–3,A). This pattern of inferior ventricular hypertrophy may in fact reflect either RVH or LVH, and
associated ECG findings must be used as an aid in
diagnosis. Posterior LVH is reflected by large negative deflections in chest leads V_1 and V_2 (Fig
3–3,B).

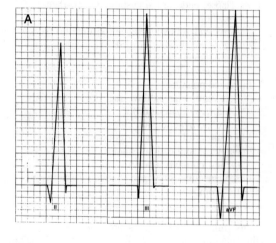

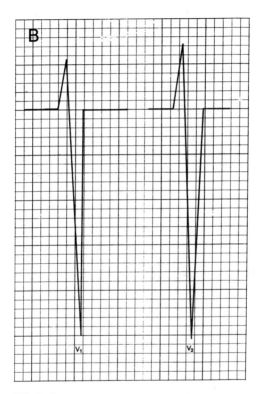

FIG 3-3.
A, "inferior" LVH pattern. **B,** "posterior" LVH pattern.

One can see from the preceding discussion that considerable experience may be required to diagnose LVH consistently. The suspicion that LVH may be present is an essential asset to accurate diagnosis.

BIVENTRICULAR HYPERTROPHY

In some conditions, both left and right ventricles are hypertrophied (see box on common causes of BVH). When that is the case, diagnostic criteria for either RVH or LVH may be modified "downward," and a diagnosis of BVH made. In this regard, when RVH is accompanied by a 7-mm R wave in aVR, usually little or no negative deflection exists in that lead. If an R wave of 4 or 5 mm in aVR is accompanied by an S wave of 13 mm, a diagnosis of BVH must be entertained. When both ventricles are hypertrophied, right *and* left precordial T wave changes are not uncommon, and large equiphasic deflections in the midprecordial leads (V_3–V_5) can be substantial—the Katz-Wachtel phenomenon (Garson, 1983).

COMMON CAUSES OF BIVENTRICULAR HYPERTROPHY

Left-to-right shunts distal to the left atrium with increased pulmonary artery pressure (VSD, PDA, etc.)

Complex CHD lesions—endocardial cushion defect, transposition of the great vessels with left ventricular outflow tract obstruction, double outlet right ventricle

---

ABNORMAL QRS CONFIGURATIONS

The initial portion of the QRS complex is due to septal depolarization proceeding from left to right, resulting in a Q wave in the left precordial leads. In some forms of congenital heart defects, the ventricular septum does not exist or is positioned abnormally. When that is the case, the Q wave deflection is affected. Under normal circumstances, the ventricular activation pattern is RS in the right precordium and qRs in the left. If the ventricles are inverted in their position (as in "corrected transposition"), the septal depolarization will occur from right to left rather than the normal left-to-right direction; this, in turn, will eliminate the q wave from the left precordial leads and transfer it to the right-sided ones. The *absence* of left precordial q waves together with a qRs pattern in the right precordium (from V_1 to V_6R depending on ventricular position) suggests the malformation of ventricular inversion. Lastly, in cases where one of the ventricles is hypoplastic or in cases where there is a single ventricle with no functional ventricular septum, Q waves may not appear in *any* of the chest leads. When that is the case, a diagnosis of single ventricle (functional or actual) may be entertained.

NOTES

NOTES

DISORDERS OF RATE AND RHYTHM

4

The heart rate is controlled normally by the sinus node. This group of cells is not the only cardiac tissue capable of spontaneous depolarization (and therefore rate control). Although the sinus node is innervated more heavily and subject to finer control than other potential cardiac pacemaker sites, atrial, junctional (or perinodal), and ventricular tissues all are able to spontaneously depolarize and control heart rate. Under physiologic conditions, however, they do so at a rate *slower* than the sinus node's. Therefore, the sinus node controls rate not because of a singular electrophysiologic property, but because it "beats other pacemaker sites to the draw." The more rapid sinus rate depolarizes the slower potential pacemakers and thereby "suppresses" them. When the sinus node slows or fails to depolarize, a slower pacemaker site *escapes* from suppression, resulting in isolated escape beats or escape rhythms. The potentially fastest pacemaker site next to the sinus node is other atrial tissue (ectopic atrial rhythm), followed by tissues around the AV node (junctional rhythm) or His-Purkinje system, and then the ventricular muscle itself (idioventricular

ARRHYTHMIA ASSOCIATIONS

PACs—infectious/inflammatory, trauma/cardiac surgery, drugs/medication, endocrine (thyroid), metabolic, neonatal

PVCs—drugs/medication, infectious/inflammatory, irritative (catheters), CNS-related, mitral valve prolapse, "developmental"

Bradycardias

  Sinus—physical conditioning, high vagal tone, increased intracranial pressure, drugs/medication, sinus node trauma/disease

  Nonsinus—same as above

  First or second degree AV block—post cardiac surgery, drugs/medication, electrolyte imbalance, myopathy, postinfectious/inflammatory

  Complete heart block—congenital, post surgery, postinfectious/inflammatory

Tachycardias

  Sinus—physiologic (anemia, fever, hypovolemia, etc.), CNS, drugs/medication, endocrine (thyroid)

  SVT—see text; dual pathways, WPW, CHD

  Atrial flutter—post cardiac surgery, myopathy, CHD

  Junctional ectopic tachycardia—post cardiac surgery

  Ventricular tachycardia—irritative (catheters), drugs/medication, trauma (surgery), postinfectious/inflammatory, hypoxemia/acidosis, electrolyte imbalance

rhythm). If one of these alternative pacemaker sites is controlling the heart at a rate *less* than a normal sinus rate, the implication is that the sinus node is not functioning properly, owing to vagal suppression, disease, drugs, trauma, or other factors (see box on Arrhythmia Associations). In other words, an ectopic escape rhythm (one with a rate slower than a sinus rhythm) is a fail-safe mechanism, *not* a hostile takeover of the physiologic norm.

Table 1–1 establishes *broad guidelines* of sinus heart rate for children from 1 day to 10 years of age. The lower limit of "normal" in older children is surrounded by question marks, for in this day of long-distance running and prepubertal athletic superstars, highly conditioned youngsters may "normally" have sinus rates of 45 to 55 bpm at rest.

Variations in heart rate are expectable during phases of respiration (Fig 4–1) and changes in vagal tone, as well as in response to metabolic changes associated with changes in:

Temperature
Activity
Catecholamine levels (anxiety, fear, endocrine disorders)
Diet

Note also that rates listed are beats per *minute*. Children normally may have short (5–10 bpm) runs of bradycardia at rates less than those listed; however, when the actual beats per *minute* are totaled, the sum will be higher than the number extrapolated from the brief interval of bradycardia.

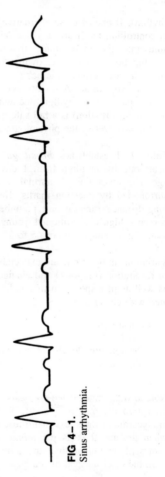

FIG 4–1.
Sinus arrhythmia.

Changes in rate and rhythm that are not physiologic provide some of the most challenging diagnostic puzzles in pediatric cardiology. These rate and rhythm disorders are overviewed briefly here. In many circumstances, however, subspecialty and subsubspecialty expertise is needed to solve the riddle.

ECTOPIC BEATS

Beats coming from an unanticipated location (ectopic) may occur early or late in a rhythm sequence. If they are *early,* they are *premature;* if they appear *late,* they are called *escape* beats, a physiologic response to slowing or discontinuation of the previous pacemaker site, as discussed above. The distinction between premature ectopic beats (Fig 4–2) and physiologic escape beats (Fig 4–3) is a critical one to make.

Premature Atrial "Contractions"

Atrial premature beats are often recognizable because a P wave with different axis and appearance from the sinus P wave is visible before the QRS complex. In addition, PACs may be nonconducted ("blocked"), causing a prolonged pause between R waves (Fig 4–4).

The atrial origin of a premature beat may be difficult to establish if conduction of the impulse through the ventricles is aberrant, giving the general appearance of a ventricular premature beat. Even in this case, P waves may be visible; also, the more premature the beat, the more aberrant the conduc-

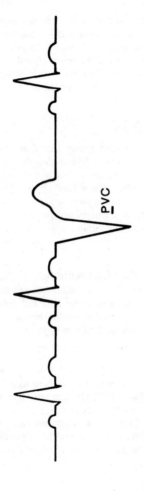

FIG 4–2.
Premature ventricular contraction.

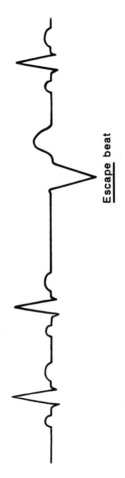

FIG 4–3.
Ventricular *escape* beat.

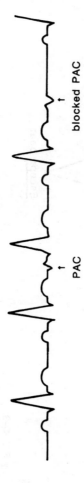

FIG 4–4.
Premature atrial contractions *(PAC)*, one of which is not conducted to the ventricle (blocked).

tion, a relationship which may tip off the origin of
the ectopic impulse (Fig 4–5).

Premature Ventricular Contractions

Ventricular premature beats usually have broader
QRS complexes (have a longer ventricular conduction time) than those associated with PACs, and fre-
quently have a T wave axis opposite in direction to
that of the QRS complex (Fig 4–6). The "compensatory pause" following the premature beat is tradi-
tionally said to be *complete* with a PVC (that is, the
interval between the two sinus beats surrounding the
PVC is *twice* the interval between two consecutive
sinus beats) as the sinus node may be unaffected by
a PVC when retrograde conduction to the atrium is
blocked at the AV node. Conversely, with PACs,
the sinus node is "reset" by the premature atrial
beat, and the compensatory pause is *incomplete* (the
interval between the two sinus beats surrounding the
PAC is less than twice the normal sinus cycle
length).

Many exceptions exist to these interpretation guidelines, however, as when the PVC starts just below
the AV node (in or near the conduction system). In
that case, the QRS complex is narrow and the T
wave virtually identical to that of the sinus beat.
Distinguishing PACs from PVCs may not be possi-
ble from surface tracings, but the following points
may help:

- Examine ectopic beats from the perspective of
  more than one lead. What may be obvious in
  lead II can be obscure in lead I (Fig 4–7).

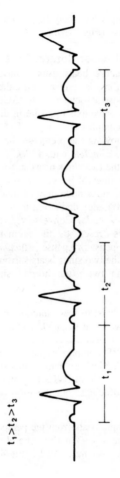

$t_1 > t_2 > t_3$

FIG 4–5.
Rate-dependent aberrancy with PACs.

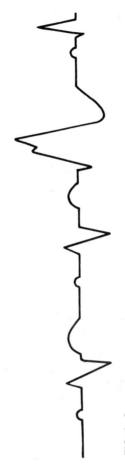

FIG 4–6.
Premature ventricular contraction.

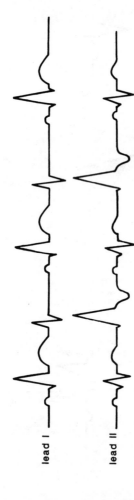

FIG 4–7.
Variation in QRS morphology with change in observation axis (lead).

- *Fusion* beats are hybrids between the sinus wave form and an ectopic beat. Fusion beats *almost* always represent combinations of the sinus beat with a *ventricular* ectopic beat. The PVC becomes incorporated into the QRS complex as it "meets" the sinus beat beyond the AV node (Fig 4–8).
- *Interpolated* beats are ectopic beats occurring within beats of sinus rhythm, without materially disturbing the basic rate mechanism. The persistence of a physiologic atrial rhythm in the presence of ectopic beats all but guarantees a subnodal ("ventricular") origin to the ectopic beats (Fig 4–9).

Ventricular ectopic beats are common in pediatric patients. When they are isolated, all have the same appearance (unifocal). They disappear with increasing heart rate, and are most often benign. Findings which *may* demand more careful attention are ventricular premature beats occurring in strings of two or more (Fig 4–10,a); ectopic beats of clearly differing morphology and relationship to the previous sinus beat (multifocal PVCs, Fig 4–10,b); PVCs occurring in patients receiving digitalis or catecholamine-like drugs; PVCs occurring together with hypokalemia or hypercapnia; or ectopic beats with varying coupling intervals but identical morphology (unless fusion occurs) called *parasystole* because the interval between ectopic beats is a multiple of the shortest interectopic "cycle length" (Fig 4–10,c).

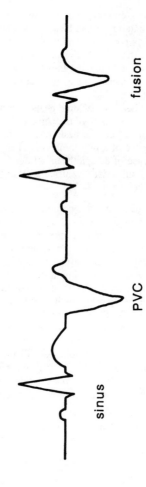

FIG 4–8.
Premature ventricular contraction (*PVC*) and *fusion* beat.

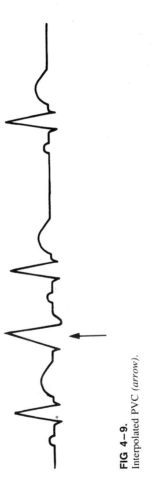

FIG 4–9.
Interpolated PVC (*arrow*).

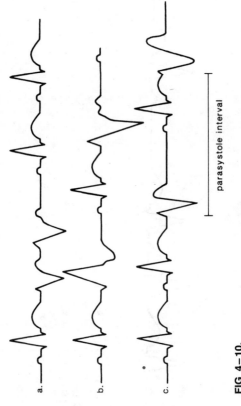

FIG 4–10.
PVCs. **a,** couplet. **b,** multifocal. **c,** parasystole (coupling interval varies).

BRADYCARDIAS (SLOW HEART RATES)

Bradycardias refer to heart rates slower than the accepted lower range of normal for sinus rate. They may be sinus or nonsinus.

Sinus Bradycardia

A sinus rate slower than the lower limit of normal heart rate for a given age is referred to as a *sinus bradycardia*. As mentioned previously, conditioned youngsters may have normal hemodynamics with a heart rate below the "accepted" lower limit of normal heart rate. This diagnosis of physiologic bradycardia must be entertained and made with caution; nevertheless, in some instances, a slow sinus rate is not pathologic.

If the sinus rate for a given age is not met consistently in a youngster who does not fulfill the fitness criteria mentioned, the implication is that sinus node function is abnormal. Sinus bradycardia may be associated with low body temperature, anesthetic drugs, β-blocking agents, and surgical or other trauma. If the sinus rate is very low and an accessory pacemaker rhythm does not take over, the implication is that the cardiac depolarization system is affected diffusely by the inciting cause, and all cardiac pacemaker sites are functioning abnormally.

Nonsinus Bradycardia

By definition, the basic rhythm is not sinus rhythm. In this circumstance, an accessory pacemaker site has taken over. The rate of depolarization of that pacemaker site is such, however, that the intrinsic heart rate does not meet the lower limit of normal for the age. In this instance, an ectopic atrial, junctional, or ventricular accessory rhythm is slower than the accepted range of normal sinus rhythm, resulting in a nonsinus bradycardia.

HEART BLOCK (AV BLOCK)

Heart block is subclassified into first, second, and third degree types.

First Degree Heart Block

In first degree heart block, the PR interval exceeds the upper limit of normal for age and heart rate (Fig 4–11). Each P wave is followed by a QRS complex, but the PR interval is prolonged.

Second Degree Heart Block

Second degree heart block is defined as intermittent nonconduction of P waves through the AV node to the ventricles. In type I second degree block (Wenckebach phenomenon), the PR interval lengthens progressively and the R-R interval shortens until a P wave is not conducted through the AV node. In this phenomenon, cycles of two or more QRS complexes are spaced apart by the nonconducted P wave (Fig 4–12). The implication of type I second degree block is AV node disease. In type II second degree AV block (rare in the pediatric population), P waves intermittently are not conducted, but without a recognizable pattern of PR interval lengthening. Type II second degree AV block most often reflects disease within the His bundle and is potentially lethal.

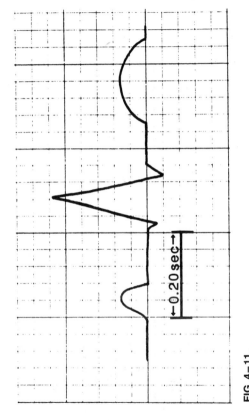

FIG 4–11.
First degree AV block.

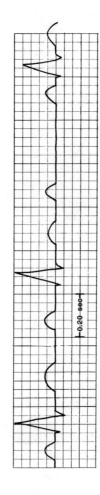

|←0.20 sec→|

FIG 4–12.
Type I second degree AV block (Wenckebach phenomenon).

Third Degree Heart Block

In third degree heart block, no relationship exists between the atrial and ventricular rates *and,* for secure diagnosis, the atrial rate exceeds the ventricular rate (Fig 4–13). The term *AV dissociation* has been used interchangeably with third degree AV block; this may lead to confusion. AV dissociation is a nonspecific term which refers to a condition due either to AV block or junctional or ventricular rhythms with a rate exceeding that of the sinus node. In AV dissociation *without diagnosable conduction block,* no relationship exists between atrial and ventricular rates, *but* the ventricular rate exceeds the atrial rate (Fig 4–14). In this type of AV dissociation, the atrial rate may be slowed to the extent that an accessory pacemaker site in the ventricle or near the AV junction takes over. When this occurs and the junctional impulse is not conducted retrograde to depolarize the atria, the P waves and QRS complexes may lose their 1:1 relationship, but the ventricular rate exceeds the atrial rate. This phenomenon allows *no* conclusions to be drawn about AV conduction; sinus node or atrial pacemaker dysfunction is the diagnosable abnormality, although true third degree heart block may coexist. In this circumstance, an occasional sinus beat may be conducted to the ventricle, giving a clue that true third degree AV block does not exist. When, in the presence of AV dissociation, the atrial rate exceeds the ventricular rate *and* the P waves are not followed regularly by a QRS complex, one may conclude that normal AV node conduction is interrupted.

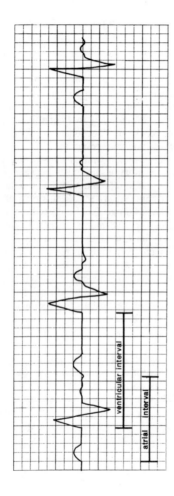

FIG 4–13.
Third degree AV block.

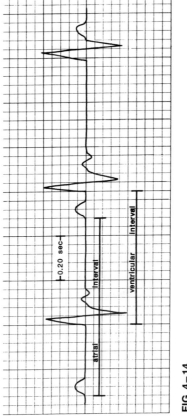

FIG 4–14.
AV dissociation. Third degree AV block is *not* a certainty.

TACHYCARDIAS (RAPID HEART RATES)

Sinus Tachycardia

Sinus rhythm with a rate exceeding the upper limit of normal for age is termed *sinus tachycardia*. Sinus tachycardia often is a physiologic response to an inciting cause. The causes include temperature elevation, high circulating catecholamine levels, a high level of autonomic tone, drugs, and any condition which increases cardiac output needs (anemia, structural heart disease, myocardial muscle dysfunction, etc.). When sinus tachycardia is diagnosed, one is obligated to search for the inciting cause.

Supraventricular Tachycardia

Subjects predisposed to SVT may have *two* AV nodal pathways for the conduction of impulses between the atria and the ventricles: one pathway, normally the more rapidly conducting route, has a long refractory period; the other pathway, normally the slow conducting route, has a shorter refractory period. In typical SVT, a PAC is conducted via the slow pathway (with the short refractory period) from atrium to ventricle anterograde; retrograde conduction from the ventricle to atrium occurs later in the cycle through the pathway with more rapid conduction, but with the longer refractory period (Akhtar, 1984). In this circumstance, the PR interval is longer than the interval between the R wave and the next P wave in the ECG tracing. This is referred to by some as the long PR, short RP pattern, and is the typical pattern of SVT in children (stylized and actual SVT tracings are shown in Fig 4–15). In some subjects, however, the pathway with the longer refractory period also has the slower

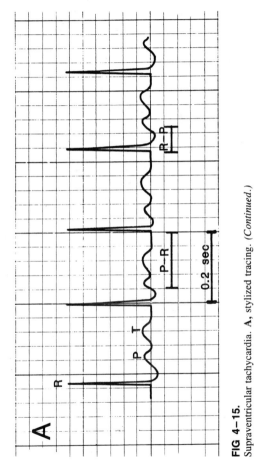

FIG 4–15.
Supraventricular tachycardia. A, stylized tracing. *(Continued.)*

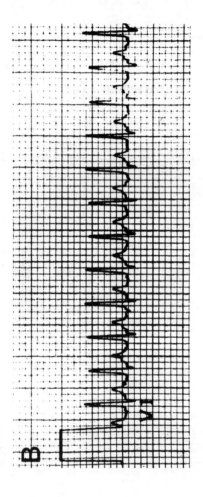

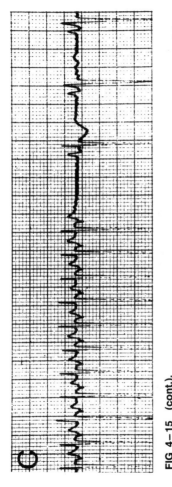

FIG 4–15 (cont.).
B, actual tracing: upright P waves, PR>RP interval. **C,** spontaneous termination of SVT: inverted P waves during tachycardia change to upright P waves following conversion to sinus rhythm.

conduction time; this pattern of SVT (short PR, long RP) is less common in children. In Wolff-Parkinson-White syndrome (WPW), an anomalous conduction pathway outside the AV node connects the atria directly with the ventricular muscle. If it is conducting, this pathway has a rapid conduction time, but a long refractory period. With nonconducting WPW pathways, rhythm is sinus and the QRS complex is normal. With an anterograde conducting pathway, impulse conduction to the ventricle may be normal (AV nodal conduction) or aberrant (WPW pathway) with a short PR interval and a wide QRS complex commencing with a *delta* wave whose axis is dependent on the site of entry of the pathway into the ventricle (Fig 4–16). Lastly, a retrograde conducting pathway predisposes the subject to a reentrant tachycardia, because two AV conduction pathways with different conduction rates and refractory periods exist—one within the AV node, and one directly between the atrium and ventricle.

In typical WPW SVT, the QRS complex is narrow and the rate is high, often exceeding 260 bpm (see Fig 4–15). In some cases (about 50%) a P wave is visible prior to each QRS complex (Gillette and Garson, 1981). With this pattern—a visible P wave, a narrow QRS complex, and a heart rate approaching 300 bpm—little question exists about the correct diagnosis. In some cases, however, the diagnosis is not straightforward. When P waves are not visible and the rate approximates 200 bpm, correct diagnosis may be difficult if conduction through the ventricles is slowed ("aberrant") (Fig 4–17). This circumstance may mimic ventricular tachycardia and be impossible to distinguish from it without invasive study.

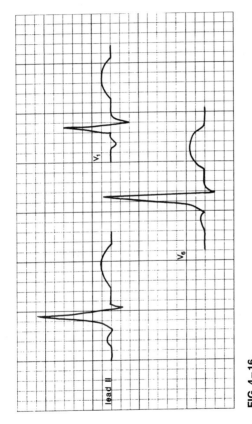

FIG 4–16.
Wolff-Parkinson-White syndrome, type b.

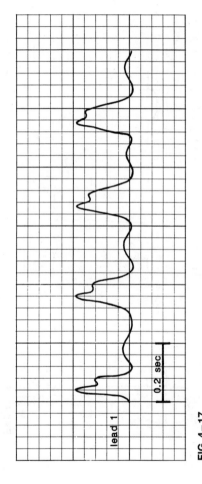

lead 1

0.2 sec

FIG 4–17.
SVT with aberrancy and nonvisible P waves.

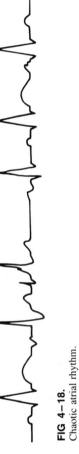

FIG 4–18.
Chaotic atrial rhythm.

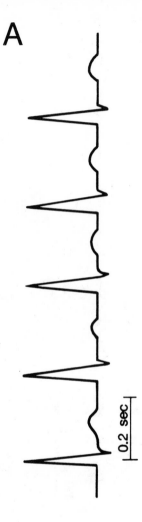

FIG 4–19.
Junctional ectopic tachycardia. A, P waves not visible. *Continued.*

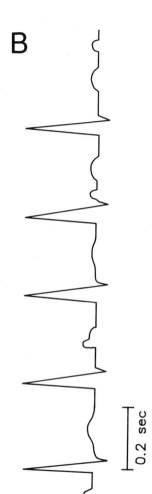

FIG 4–19 (cont.).
B, a slower, atrial sinus rhythm with AV dissociation is present.

A number of other atrial tachyarrhythmias exist:

- Chaotic atrial rhythm—atrial discharges from a number of sites in the atria or junctional region intermittently capture the ventricle, resulting in an irregularly irregular rhythm with P waves of differing morphology and a varying PR interval (Fig 4–18)
- Junctional ectopic tachycardia—this difficult-to-treat rhythm disorder occurs most commonly in the postoperative period and is characterized by a narrow complex, moderately rapid rate pattern without detectable P waves or (Fig 4–19) with AV dissociation.
- Atrial flutter—the atrial discharge is rapid and rhythmic, often inscribing a sawtoothed pattern in some leads, and commonly blocked at a 2:1 or 3:1 ratio (Fig 4–20)
- Atrial fibrillation—an uncommon rhythm in pediatrics, diagnosable by the irregularly irregular rate without discernible P waves on the ECG tracing (Fig 4–21)

Ventricular Tachycardia

Ventricular tachycardia is characterized typically by rates lower than those of SVT and is often associated with a wide QRS complex resulting from slowed, aberrant conduction through the ventricles. When the ventricular focus lies outside the conduction system, much of the transmission of the electrical impulse occurs through the heart muscle and, predictably, slurs the QRS complex. In VT, anterograde P wave conduction is not present, and the configuration of the QRS and T waves in selected leads is typical (Fig 4–22).

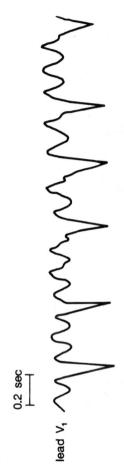

FIG 4–20.
Atrial flutter.

lead V₁

0.2 sec

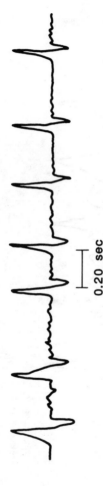

0.20 sec

FIG 4–21.
Atrial fibrillation.

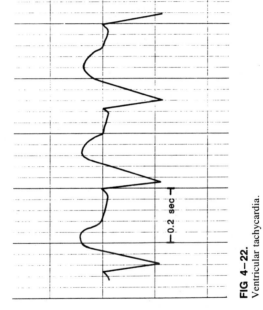

FIG 4–22.
Ventricular tachycardia.

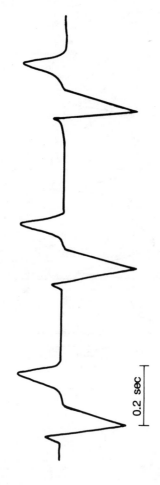

FIG 4–23.
Hyperkalemia.

0.2 sec

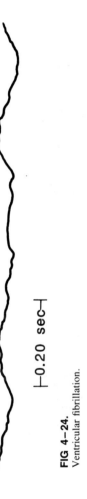

├─0.20 sec─┤

FIG 4–24.
Ventricular fibrillation.

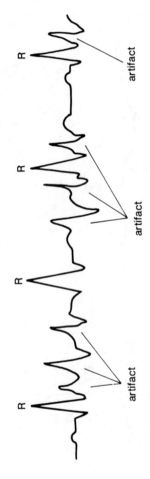

FIG 4–25.
ECG artifacts.

Ventricular tachycardia must be distinguished from SVT with aberrant conduction (see above) and from the QRS-T pattern of hyperkalemia, a pattern which may mimic VT closely (Fig 4–23). In hyperkalemia patterns, the basic rate changes are not abrupt, as they are with the transition from sinus rhythm to VT; in fact, tachycardia, as defined, may not be present at all. In hyperkalemia, the primary abnormality is one of conduction.

Ventricular fibrillation is a catastrophic event in pediatrics, as in adult medicine. The subtypes of *fine* and *coarse* VF affect the treatment approach, but not the deleterious effects of this rhythm on the circulation (Fig 4–24).

ARTIFACTS

Artifacts may confuse the interpretation of ECGs, especially as viewed on monitors in the intensive care unit (ICU) setting. The detection of ECG artifact is as much an art as it is a science (Stanger et al., 1977). A wide variety of factors may account for ECG artifact, including electrical interference, chest percussion, hiccups, and seizures (Fig 4–25). A hint to aid in distinguishing artifact from tachyarrhythmia is careful observation of the QRS-T complex; with artifact, the appearance of the QRS-T complex is *regular,* and multiple, bizarre baseline variations are interspersed with the regular rhythm. It is helpful as well to change the lead of observation in an effort to distinguish the true QRS-T complexes from the artifactual deflections.

NOTES

IMPLANTABLE
CARDIAC
PACEMAKERS

5

Cardiac pacing is becoming an increasingly common aspect of pediatric cardiology. Intrinsic impulse generation abnormalities or conduction tissue disease, together with injury to the sinus or AV node during cardiac surgery, are the usual causes for pacemaker implantation. Specific indications for permanent cardiac pacing include:

- Sinus node disease or dysfunction.
- Congenital third degree AV block with heart rates usually under 45 bpm and circulatory congestion *or* at higher rates with coexistent structural congenital heart disease.
- Surgical heart block or sinus node injury.
- Rhythm disorders requiring treatment with medications that cause either severe bradycardia or heart block or both.

A *cursory* review of pacemaker nomenclature and technology is given here to aid the reader in analysis of ECG tracings in which a pacemaker plays a part.

LEADS

Activation of the heart occurs through an electrical connection between the pacemaker generator and the myocardial tissue. The connecting device is referred to as a *pacemaker lead*. Two general types are available:

1. The *epicardial* lead is sewn directly to the epicardium.
2. The *transvenous* lead tip is fixed to the endocardium following venous insertion and advancement into the heart.

As a general statement, epicardial leads are used in small patients, in whom venous access and endocardial placement are problematic. They are also used in some subjects with major congenital cardiac malformations allowing communication between the right and left sides of the heart; the epicardial lead is used to eliminate the risk of clot embolization from an endocardial lead to the systemic circulation. Epicardial leads have the disadvantage of requiring thoracotomy for placement. Also, the electrical conductivity threshold is usually higher for an epicardial than an endocardial lead; the higher threshold requires a stronger or longer stimulation spike, which in turn may drain the generator battery prematurely.

Endocardial leads placed following venous introduction are used increasingly in pediatrics. Typically, a branch of the subclavian vein beneath the clavicle is isolated and cannulated. The lead tip is advanced under fluoroscopic control into the right heart, where it is "fixed" to the atrial or ventricular wall by one of a number of tip configurations. The lead is placed preferentially in the appendage of the atrium, or the apex of the ventricle, as indicated by the physiologic circumstance. Slack is introduced into the system to allow for some growth and lead elongation. Transvenous leads require less stimulation energy than epicardial leads, but are more prone to dislodgment.

PACEMAKER GENERATORS
Nomenclature
Pacemaker generators are referred to typically by three initials, listed in sequence— $X_1X_2X_3$:

X_1 refers to the chamber *paced:*
   A = atrium
   V = ventricle
   D = dual, or both atrium and ventricle

X_2 refers to the chamber *sensed,* again, A, V, and D

X_3 refers to the *mode* of pacemaker function, following sensing:
   I = inhibited
   T = triggered
   D = dual, may be triggered or inhibited

Mode of Operation
Examples of generator types are VVI, VAT, and DDD.

Single Chamber
VVI pacemakers pace and sense the ventricles, and the generator function is *i*nhibited following sensing

of a ventricular impulse. With VVI pacemakers, a single lead may be attached epicardially or endocardially to the ventricle. If a ventricular impulse is sensed, the unit is inhibited (turned off). If no impulse is sensed in a specified interval, the pacemaker discharges and captures the ventricle.

Two Chamber

VAT pacemakers pace the ventricle, sense the atrium, and are triggered following sensing of the atrial impulse. These pacemakers coordinate atrial and ventricular contractions. They require, however, that atrial activation and conduction be normal; they would be inappropriate for use in someone with a slow, junctional rhythm.

Physiologic

DDD pacemakers are connected to both atrial and ventricular leads. They have a range of capabilities. These units can act as VAT or VVI generators by programming the pacemaker variables appropriately; however, they can also act as standby or control units sensing all electrical cycle events and contributing only what is "needed." Accordingly, the DDD unit can be programmed to pace the atria at a rate of 90 bpm and, following a 160-ms AV delay, discharge the ventricles after each atrial beat. If the atria intrinsically start to discharge at a rate over 90 bpm, however, the atrial stimulus will be inhibited; the ventricle will still be stimulated 160 ms after the atrial beat, unless intrinsic AV conduction and ventricular discharge occur more rapidly than that (Fig 5–1). These pacemakers provide a wide range of pacing capabilities, but are associated with a wide range of complications and malfunctions as well. Their use in pediatrics is limited.

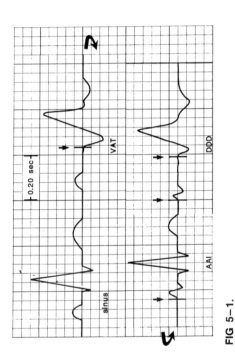

FIG 5–1.
Physiologic (*DDD*) pacemaker functioning in atrially triggered (*VAT*), atrially inhibited (*AAI*), and dual chamber pacing (*DDD*) modes.

Rate-Responsive

A new generation of pacemakers is referred to as *rate-responsive*. These units use one of several types of monitoring systems to increase pacing rate when a physiologic need arises. The units are connected typically to the ventricle and set with a lower rate limit. Their circuitry includes a device to monitor some physiologic variable, such as motion or ventilatory minute volume. When the pacemaker unit senses an increase in the monitored variable, the pacemaker rate is increased in a programmed way to match the physiologic need. These units are promising and still undergoing developmental modifications.

Complications

Pacemaker units currently are small, powered by lithium batteries with projected body lives of 4 to 9 years, and quite reliable. Many pacemaker variables, such as rate, impulse strength and duration, sensitivity, refractory period, and AV delay are programmable and can be interrogated by telemetry. However, when potential complications such as infection, lead fracture or dislodgment, generator failure, and unit malfunction are added together, one must anticipate system modification or adjustment on average every 3 to 4 years.

NOTES

NOTES

REFERENCES

Ahnve S: Correction of the QT interval for heart rate: Review of different formulas and the use of Bazett's formula in myocardial infarction. *Am Heart J* 1985; 109:568.

Akhtar M: Supraventricular tachycardias—electrophysiologic mechanisms, diagnosis, and pharmacologic therapy, in Josephson ME, Wellens HJJ (eds): *Tachycardia—Mechanisms, Diagnosis, Treatment,* Philadelphia, Lea & Febiger, 1984, pp 137–140.

Garson A Jr (ed): *The Electrocardiogram in Infants and Children: A Systematic Approach,* Philadelphia, Lea & Febiger, 1983 pp 108–110.

Gillette PC, Garson A Jr (eds): *Pediatric Arrhythmias: Electrophysiology and Pacing.* Philadelphia, WB Saunders, 1990.

Marriott, HJL (ed): *Practical Electrocardiography,* ed 8. Baltimore, Williams & Wilkins Co, 1983, p 81.

Schwartz PJ, Montemerlo M, Facchini M, et al: The QT interval throughout the first 6 months of life: A prospective study, *Circulation* 1982; 66:496.

Schwartz PJ, Periti M, Malliani A: The long QT syndrome. *Am Heart J* 1975; 89:378.

Stanger P, Lister G Jr, Silverman NH, et al: Electrocardiographic monitor artifacts in a neonatal intensive care unit. *Pediatrics* 1977; 60:689.

APPENDIX A

Characteristic ECG Patterns in Congenital Heart Disease (CHD)

CHD Category	Axis	P Wave	QRS	Other
Left-to-right shunts				
PDA				Left precordial ST/T abnormalities
ASD	+90–150		rSR' in right precordium	
VSD or DORV		LAE............. RAE.............	.LVH............. .RVH.............	.with high flow .with high pulmonary vascular resistance or PS
AV canal (endocardial cushion defect)	−20 to −150	(P and QRS as with VSD)		Counterclockwise vector loop
Obstructive lesions				
PS	+90–280	±RAE	RVH	ECG sensitive index of severity
AS		±LAE	±LVH	ECG *not* a sensitive index of severity
Aortic coarctation				
In newborn	Right axis	±RAE	RVH	
After 6–12 months	Left axis	±LAE	±LVH	

Condition	QRS axis	Atrial enlargement	Ventricular hypertrophy	Comments
Anomalous drainage of pulmonary veins with obstruction	+90–210	RAE	RVH	qR pattern in right precordium
Right-to-left shunts Tetralogy of Fallot	+90–180	RAE	RVH	Early transition from right to left precordial pattern
Tricuspid atresia	*−30 to −150*	RAE	LVH	*If great vessels transposed, QRS axis may be positive*
Pulmonary atresia	Right axis	RAE	**	**Right ventricular forces depend on right ventricular size
Ebstein's anomaly of tricuspid valve	Right axis	RAE	WPW pattern common	
Transposition of the great vessels	Right axis			
Truncus arteriosus	. . . . most often normal as newborn.			
Miscellaneous Anomalous origin of left coronary artery				. . . . . normal for newborn. . . . . . ischemia or myocardial infarction pattern
Asplenia/polysplenia syndrome				atrial axis anomalies + RVH

APPENDIX B

LIST OF ABBREVIATIONS

AS   aortic stenosis
ASD   atrial septal defect
AV   atrioventricular
bpm   beats per minute
BVH   biventricular hypertrophy
CHD   congenital heart disease
CNS   central nervous system
ECG   electrocardiogram
JET   junctional ectopic tachycardia
LAE   left atrial enlargement
LVH   left ventricular hypertrophy
PAC   premature atrial contraction
PDA   patent ductus arteriosus
PS   pulmonic stenosis
PVC   premature ventricular contraction
QT_c corrected QT interval
RAE   right atrial enlargement
RVH   right ventricular hypertrophy
SBE   subacute bacterial endocarditis
SVT   supraventricular tachycardia
VF   ventricular fibrillation
VSD   ventricular septal defect
VT   ventricular tachycardia
WPW   Wolff-Parkinson-White syndrome

INDEX

Q

Sinus node, 45
Sinus tachycardia, 68
Spontaneous depolarization, 45
Supraventricular tachycardia, 68–78

T

T wave
   characteristics of, 12
   in left ventricular hypertrophy, 36
   in right ventricular hypertrophy, 34–35
Tachycardia
   associated disorders of, 46
   sinus, 68
   supraventricular, 68–78
Third degree AV heart block, 65–67
Transvenous lead, 90
Two chamber pacemakers, 92

V

VAT pacemakers, 92
Ventricular contractions, premature. *see* Premature
   ventricular contraction
Ventricular depolarization, 7–12. *see also* QRS
   complex
Ventricular ectopic beats, 57
Ventricular escape beat, 51
Ventricular fibrillation, 83, 85
Ventricular hypertrophy
   abnormal QRS configurations and, 41
   of both left and right ventricles, 40
   causes of, 34, 40
   left, 36–40